Destress

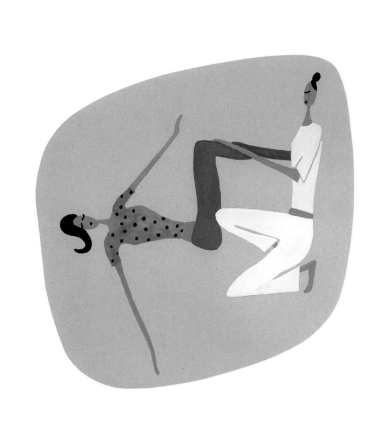

Destress

100 natural ways to relax

Carol Morley & Liz Wilde

Time Warner Books

WARNER BOOKS
An AOL Time Warner Company

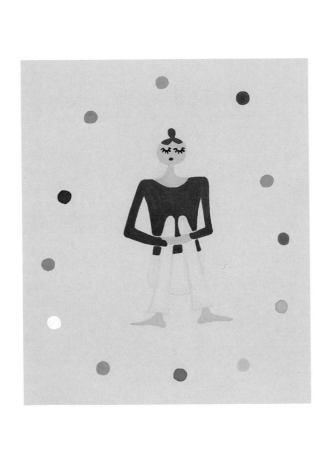

introduction

Once upon a time, stress was the body's warning system to either fight or flee from aggressors (think wild animals and unfriendly neighbors), making it essential for staying alive. Now stress is more likely to be a long-term reaction to the faster pace of life (think job security, relationships, or just fitting everything into a day). Short-term stress can be exciting, but research shows that the over-production of hormones caused by long-term stress can upset the mind and body, causing everything from indigestion to serious illnesses. We can't stop our body's natural response to stress, but we can learn how to cope with it better. This little book tells you how.

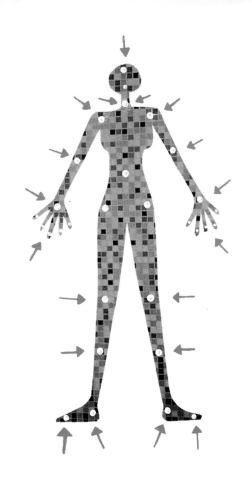

contents

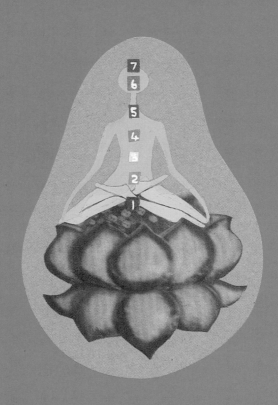

chapter 1

Stress solutions

1 **Yoga has been around for 5,000 years and, although its many famous fans have helped it become hip, its benefits remain constant.** The poses aim to bring your mind, body, and breathing together as one, which not only improves posture and physical health, but brings you a sense of inner calm. Yoga may not burn fat, but the challenging positions will tone up traditionally flabby areas such as stomach, bottom, and thighs. And if you choose the more dynamic ashtanga yoga (also known as power yoga), expect a seriously sweaty workout which will reshape your body better than any step class.

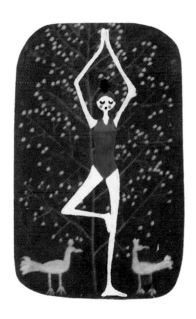

2 **Exercise is the ultimate stress solution.** Not only does it stimulate the body's pituitary gland to release tension and give you a natural high, it also tires you out so you sleep better no matter how much your brain is racing. Research also shows that regular exercise makes you less tense and better able to cope with stress.

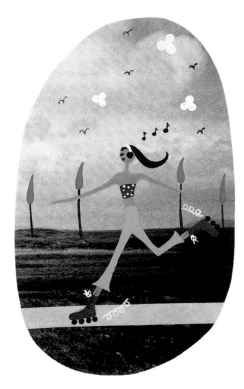

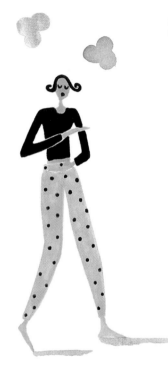

3 **Known as "meditation in motion," tai chi concentrates on slow, flowing movements to relieve stress and strengthen the body.** Unlike most martial arts, people practice tai chi for health and relaxation rather than self defense, and it's not aerobic, so don't do it to lose weight. What you will get is a stronger, more flexible body and improved posture. And the gentle movements have also been shown to relax the muscles and nervous system. Cheap and easy to start (all you need is loose clothing and a pair of flat-heeled shoes or socks), it's important to find a good teacher, so ask for references before you commit yourself to a course.

14

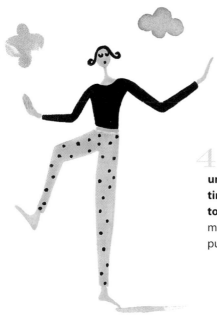

4 **You may feel exhausted, but unless you've given your body time to slow down, you won't go to sleep.** Listen to soothing music, read a book, or meditate to put your body in snooze mode.

5 **Life is getting faster, which means we have less time to do the things we should.** Like eat regularly. Skipping lunch and surviving on fast food will greatly affect your mind and body. But making time to eat a balanced diet at regular mealtimes will ensure your body remains healthy and able to cope during stressful times.

6 **Avoid eating three to four hours before bedtime,** and if you must late-night snack, eat sleep-easy foods like tuna, avocado, or a banana. And avoid late-night take-out meals, as many contain MSG, a chemical that raises adrenaline levels.

7 **Don't drink tea or coffee after 5pm,** and drop your hot chocolate habit, as chocolate will wake you up. Instead, calm down with a cup of chamomile tea to soothe you.

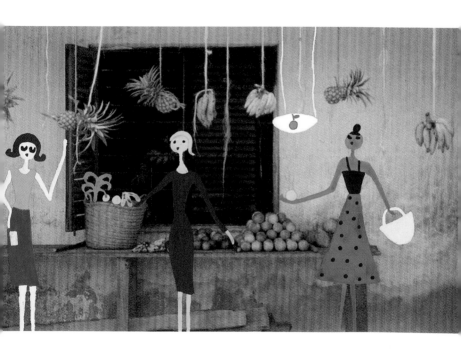

8 **Are you getting enough sleep, or do you spend your days exhausted?** Too little sleep can cause headaches, mood swings, irritability, and even weepiness. Add a little stress to the situation, and we're talking serious depression.

9 **To ensure your day ends in dreamland: Start exercising and you'll sleep more deeply.** All it takes is a brisk walk for 30 minutes three times a week, but don't exert yourself too near bedtime or you'll be too over-excited to go to sleep.

10 **Research shows that lavender oil can be just as effective as sleeping pills,** so put a few drops on your pillow or into a warm (not hot) bath before bedtime.

11 **Keep your bedroom cool (but not cold) at night,** as a drop in body temperature ensures deep sleep.

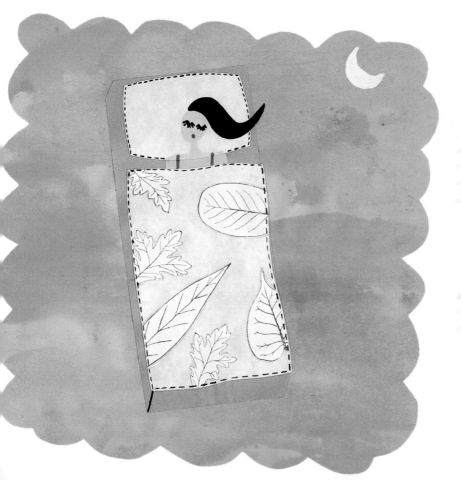

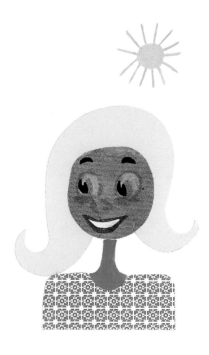

20

12 Learn to think positively and you can look forward to a longer and happier life. Evidence shows that when you feel negative about life's events, you're more likely to suffer stress, depression, and even illness. But positive thinkers can cope with just about anything. Thought patterns are learned throughout life, so if you've picked up some pessimism along the way, try a little rebalancing last thing at night. Ponder on the positive and your subconscious will soak it up while you sleep.

13 Avoid nicotine and cut down on caffeine (at most, drink three cups of tea or coffee a day), as these mimic your body's response to stressful situations. The result? A double dose of stress.

14 **Both vitamin C and B complex are depleted during stressful times,** as they're used in the production of adrenaline. Vitamin B is also used to metabolize those good old comforters alcohol and sugary foods, and a deficiency will make you more irritable than ever. If this sounds familiar, increase your intake of green vegetables, fresh fruit, nuts, seeds, and dried fruit for vitamin B, and citrus fruits (especially kiwi) to replace vitamin C. Or reach for the supplements until life slows down.

15 **Feeling unbalanced?** Color therapists believe our bodies are made up of seven main energy centers called chakras which are directly associated with and affected by a specific color. Although not part of the physical body, they link the energy fields surrounding us to the body and are responsible for our physical, mental, and spiritual health. Physical illness can start when one or more chakras become weak, but a therapist will use the correct color to positively manipulate your energy systems and restore balance.

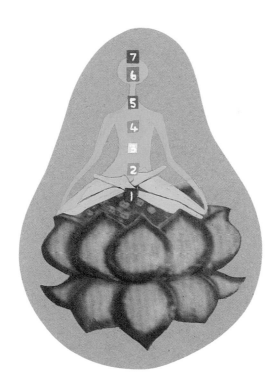

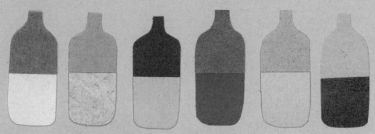

16 **The color you're drawn to says a lot about your present state of mind.** At times of stress, surround yourself with calming blues and greens which help lower blood pressure and reduce your heart rate.

Turquoise—You're optimistic, intuitive, and good at relating to others, as you have a natural empathy.

Yellow—You're feeling full of joy and optimism, probably because of a recent boost to your confidence.

Green—You're generous, especially relating to issues of the heart, but friends can think you're a little bit spaced out.

Blue—You're feeling peaceful, secure, and relaxed with an inner serenity.

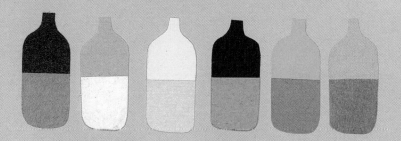

Orange—You're creative, spontaneous, and feeling good about life at the moment.

Red—You're passionate and temperamental, but also courageous and full of energy.

17 **Plants were the first medicine,** and today herbalism is again big business thanks to our love of all things holistic.

Top tablets to take in times of stress include:

Kava kava—instantly relaxing

Passionflower—relieves stress-fuelled insomnia

Skullcap—relaxes exhausted nerves

Ginseng—increases your body's ability to cope with a stressful life.

18 **Fans of flotation describe it as the deepest rest they've ever had,** so why does lying in a foot of buoyant water in a sound- and light-proof tank feel so good? Let us count the ways. First, the feeling of total weightlessness frees the brain and body from gravity, a cause of health problems. This cues the release of major energy and brainpower, plus an instant soothing of aches and pains. A float also increases the secretion of happy-making hormones while reducing the stress-related ones. And, with no outside interruption (noise or change of temperature), you're able to relax so deeply that an hour of floating is said to have the restorative effect of four hours' sleep.

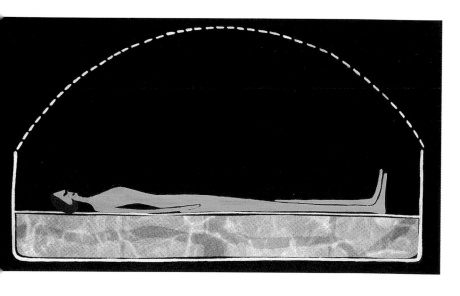

19 **One of the fastest-growing alternative therapies, Reiki is said to balance the body,** and a session can be pain-relieving, relaxing, or energizing, depending on what your body needs to feel. Reiki is literally hands-on healing, and you can expect a practitioner to place her hands on different parts of your body for up to ten minutes at a time. Especially good for relaxation and immune-system-related problems, the term Reiki means the free flow of universal energy, and, to become a practitioner, you must first learn how to open up your own healing energy force. Problems like painful joints and muscle strain can also be treated and you'll feel a deep warmth and even tingling during your treatment. Lie back and feel the force.

20 **Yet another reason to soak in, smooth on, or simply smell relaxing aromatherapy oils,** sniffing an essential oil will automatically increase inhalation, which slows down your breathing so you'll instantly feel less stressed. And the extra oxygen rush also relaxes you as it moves around your muscles.

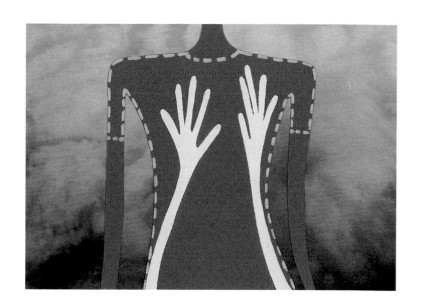

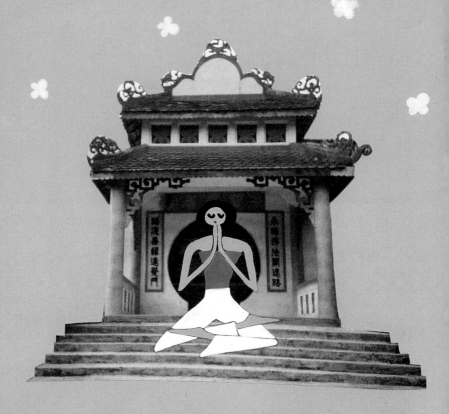

chapter 2

Destress your mind

21 Meditating regularly can seriously reduce your stress levels. Make that the transcendental type and you can expect even deeper relaxation. Transcendental meditation is said to be up to eight times more beneficial to your health than other meditation techniques. Tuition consists of a one-hour session where you are given a mantra to repeat over and over as you sit quietly. Follow-up classes fine-tune your technique. You must then meditate for 20 minutes twice a day and the aim is to reach a state of "pure consciousness" where you are neither repeating the mantra nor thinking other thoughts.

To try meditation all by yourself, sit in a quiet place where you won't be interrupted (unplug the phone) and turn down the lights/close the curtains. Make sure you're comfortable and then start to imagine each part of your body relaxing. Begin with your scalp and work down to your toes, while mentally repeating some neutral thought (try a color or cloudless sky). Concentrate on your breathing and, when thoughts break through the calm, just let them come and go. After 15 minutes, open your eyes and sit quietly for a few minutes before getting up and continuing with your ordinary day.

22 **Soothing sounds can reduce stress, lower blood pressure, and even ease pain.** Research has found that the right sounds prompt your brain to release a hormone that helps control the production of stress-inducing adrenaline. And, just like exercise, upbeat music can encourage your brain to release mood-improving endorphins. So, next time you need to be comforted, look through your CD collection for the perfect cure.

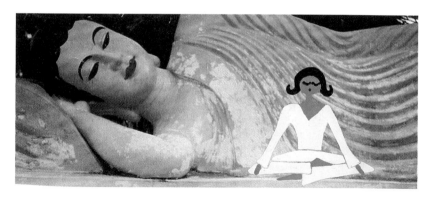

23 **Feeling tearful? Want to roll up into a ball and stay that way?** Don't lock yourself away and wallow in misery. Loving friends and family are your support network and will make you feel less isolated and depressed. And don't forget your very best friend—you! Instead of being your own worst enemy, be as nice to yourself as you are to your other friends.

24 **Know your limits and be realistic.** Don't set impossible goals (lose ten pounds in a week/learn fluent Spanish for your vacation) or you're destined to fail. And tackle big tasks one step at a time. If it all seems too much, figure out your priorities before you begin.

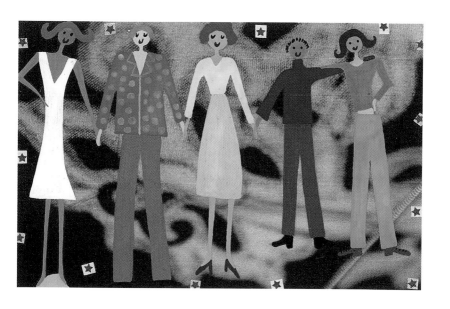

25 **Imagine you're lying on a deserted beach listening to the lapping of ocean waves and your mind will think it's on vacation.** Visualization Therapy was devised by an American radiotherapist who recognized the power of the mind when treating cancer patients. He believed (correctly) that we can fight illness and control stress with the power of our imaginations. Try it for yourself. Lie back and think of a restful scene (remember your last visit to the beach?) and focus on feeling the sun on your skin and hearing the sea splashing until all other thoughts have vanished.

26 **Feeling drained of all energy?** Then treat yourself to a (guilt-free) day in bed. Read, talk to friends on the phone, watch TV, listen to music, eat your favorite foods, or just lie there and relax.

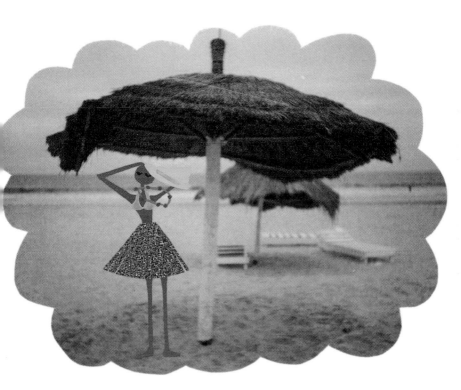

27 **Watching fish swimming in a tank is said to deeply relax the mind.** Install your own mini-aquarium at home, or visit a public one. Then sit back and chill out.

28 **Instead of worrying what everyone else is thinking, concentrate on what you're thinking instead.** You can control one, but no amount of worry will change the other.

29 **Change the things that you can change, and then learn to accept the things you can't.** No one is perfect, so don't even begin to compare yourself unfavorably with your older sister/talented friend/Cindy Crawford. Remember, your best is good enough.

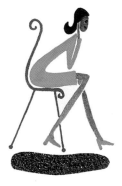

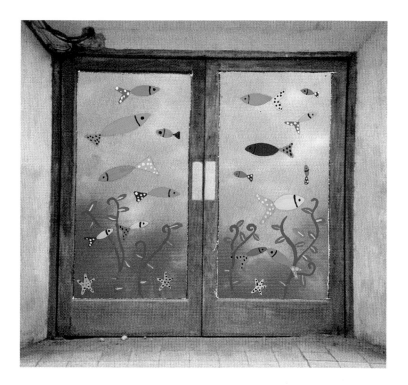

30 **When you're feeling depressed, phone your happiest friend.** It's good to talk—and even better to listen. Good relationships need good communication, and listening to your friends and family instead of interrupting their every sentence is a start. Remember, when you listen to someone, it makes them feel great. And they'll be much more likely to listen to you later!

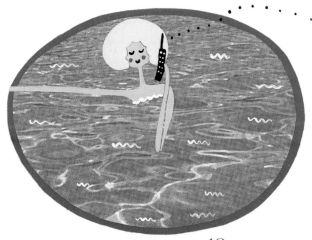

31 You're not perfect, so don't even try to be. The next time you end the day feeling guilty because you haven't been able to do everything on your wish list, repeat this less-stress mantra until you lose that feeling of helplessness.

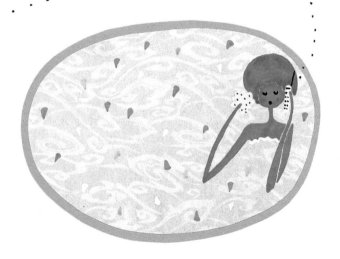

41

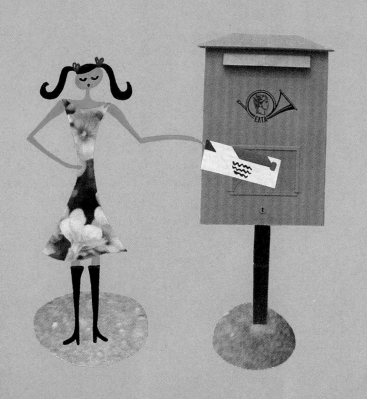

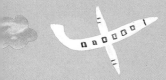

32 **Repair a troubled mind by writing down your worries.** Expressing your feelings on paper will release their intensity, making room for more positive ones in your head. Storing up anger means serious stress, which may lead to an unfortunate explosion. If you can't face a confrontation, write your thoughts down in a letter and send them off to the other person. This will help you to release negative emotions.

33 **Everyone makes mistakes. Learn from them and then move on.** But don't forget to apologize—there's nothing worse than someone who won't take responsibility for his own blunders. If, after all that humility, you need a self-confidence boost, write a list of your most recent achievements and put them on your refrigerator for regular reading.

34 **Medical experts say that holding spiritual beliefs can help strengthen your own healing capabilities.** But simply accepting there may be something bigger than ourselves allows us to let go of what we can't control. Indeed, trying to control everything is as stressful as it gets.

35 **Stuck at work with too many tasks to tackle?** Then take time to go outdoors for some fresh air, preferably somewhere green. Sit in a quiet place and concentrate on listening to your heartbeat. Close your eyes and breathe slowly and deeply, filling your lungs from the very bottom. Imagine a stream of clear water flowing over your head and through your body, collecting and cleaning out all the tension of the day. Then imagine you have roots that are growing into the ground beneath you. As you relax, your perspective will change and those tasks will now seem simpler.

36 **Learn to say no.** An unexpected question can make you feel pressurized to respond with a positive answer. The result? You take on more than you can cope with, along with soaring stress levels. Instead, trust your gut reaction and act on it. Do you feel positive or get that familiar sinking feeling? And, when it comes to saying no, do it without hundreds of excuses and without feeling guilty. You're refusing the request, not the person.

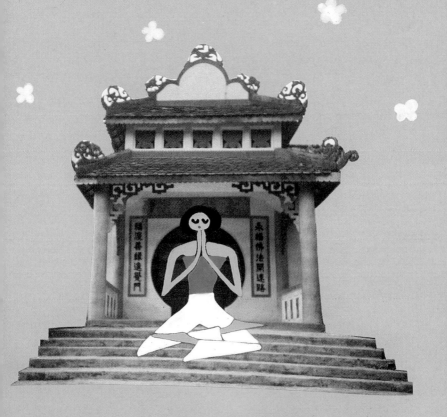

37 **Adopt the Buddhist practice of always living in the present.** Whatever you're doing—eating, walking, waiting—in whatever environment—rain, sun, snow—concentrate on the moment. The aim of this "mindfulness" is to stop your mind from wandering so that it can be at peace. If you do everything this way, you won't be able to rush things or do more than one task at a time.

38 **Remember, stress is within your control.** Behind most stressful situations is fear (you'll make a fool of yourself/no one will talk to you). Face the fear and you'll get rid of your stress.

39 **Remember, life is 10% what happens to you, and 90% how you react to it.** The choice is yours. Sometimes things are less problematic than they seem.

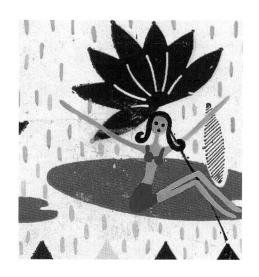

40 **Nothing in nature can hurt us when we're happy and in harmony,** claimed Dr. Edward Bach, creator of Bach Flower Remedies, back in the 1930s. He believed that conventional medicine could only bring temporary relief and didn't treat deeper emotional problems which if left unchecked could lead to more serious illnesses later. Using his medical skills,

Dr. Bach classified seven major emotional groups:

- *Fear*
- *Uncertainty*
- *Lack of interest in present circumstances*
- *Loneliness*
- *Over-sensitivity*
- *Despondency and despair*
- *Over-concern for the welfare of others.*

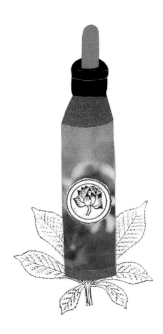

Dr. Bach then subdivided these into a total of 38 negative states of mind and formulated a plant-based remedy to treat each one. Particularly popular with stressed-out models and celebrities, Bach Flower Remedies are used around the world to restore emotional balance.

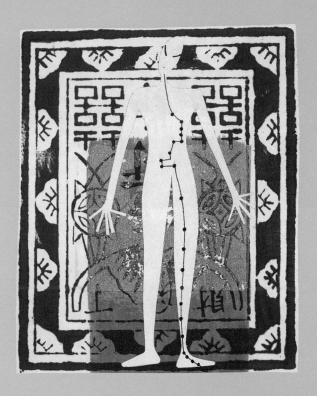

chapter 3

Destress your body

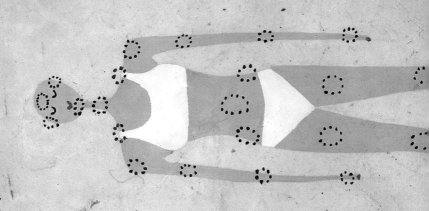

41 If you're feeling stressed, look at your body. Chances are you're all clenched up, so take time out to do these simple exercises:

- Unclench your fists and let your hands hang loosely by your sides.
- Uncross your arms and legs.
- Rotate your ankles, first one way and then the other.
- Shake your arms and legs vigorously.

42 Try this simple self-relaxation technique the next time you're stuck on a bus. Close your eyes and begin

43 **If your body regularly ends the day aching,** chances are you need Alexander Technique lessons to reduce stress and tension. The Technique's aim is to help you regain the natural poise you had as a child and thus relieve the aches and pains caused by holding yourself incorrectly. But bad habits take a lifetime to learn, and forgetting them is no overnight job, so sign up for between 15 and 25 sessions. Not cheap, but not only will you get rid of your backache, your body will look taller and leaner than before and, as an added bonus, a session feels like the most relaxing massage you've ever had.

breathing deeply, inhaling through your nose and out of your mouth. When you feel more relaxed, mentally scan your body for tension. When you find it, the next time you take a breath, as you exhale feel the breath relaxing the part of your body that's tense.

44 Lying in bed with a hyperactive mind and no chance of sleep? Starting at your forehead, work down your body, tensing each area tightly before relaxing it. Really scrunch up your face, make tight fists, and clench your bottom. By the time you reach your toes, your body will be exhausted and your mind more peaceful.

45 Feeling healthy will help you beat stress, so don't ignore long-term troubles like a bad back or bloated stomach. Cure them and you'll feel calmer in mind and body.

46 Don't eat when you're stressed. Do something relaxing and save your meal until your stomach has stopped churning.

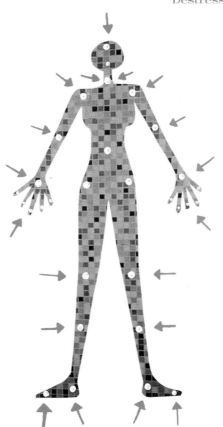

47 **Massage loosens tight muscles, relaxes your mind and body,** and research says it also decreases levels of the stress hormone cortisol. So use any excuse to have one, especially if you've been exercising regularly and deserve a reward. A massage before activity warms up muscles to prevent injury, and, after exercise, will decrease lactic acid build-up in your muscles to prevent that stiff feeling the next morning. It may even speed up your body's recovery from an injury by increasing blood flow to the area. But if you've booked a massage after training, think of your therapist and take a shower before the stroking starts.

48 **Don't eat on the run,** as this puts extra pressure on your digestion which already has a hard time during stressful situations. No matter how busy you are, sit down and savor every mouthful. Eat regularly, but don't eat just because it's lunchtime. If you don't feel hungry, wait until you do.

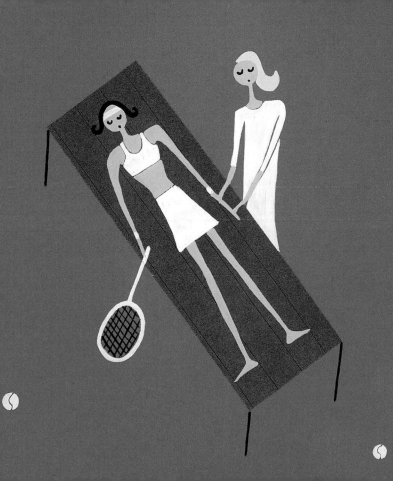

49 **Originating from China, acupuncture is an increasingly popular way to treat body organs and functions.** Fine needles are inserted into the energy channels in your body (known as meridians) to balance and restore health. The treatment is completely bloodless and mostly painless, and is successful in helping stress-related problems such as muscular pain, migraines, and headaches. First check that your acupuncturist uses disposable needles to ensure the best hygiene.

50 **Every part of your body is reflected in your feet.** A reflexologist works on "gritty" areas to massage away stress-related problems.

You can try this at home:

1. To relieve a headache, apply pressure to the pads of your fingers with the opposite hand.

2. Feel the fleshy area of your palm where your thumb meets your wrist until you find a sore point. This is your adrenal gland acupressure point. Gentle rubbing in circular movements will relax your whole body.

3. Massage your temples to relieve tension and relax your mind.

4. Pinch the area either side of the bridge of your nose to soothe a headache. Gently massage around the eye sockets to ease tension.

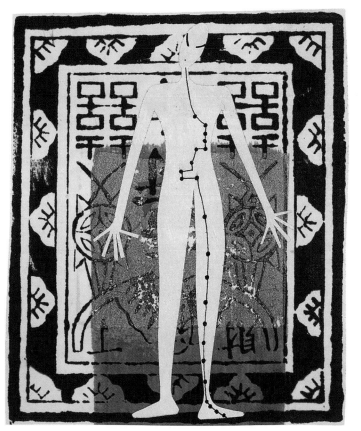

51 During acupuncture, a herb called moxa or mugwort is sometimes burned on the tip of each needle. This makes heat travel downward and warm the acupressure point, making it more receptive to treatment. And more importantly, the gentle heat feels super-soothing and relaxing on a stressed body.

52 Do-It-Yourself Massage
Most stress gets stored around your neck and lower back, so loosen up with these easy moves:

PURE MOXA

1. Place your hand over the top of your opposite shoulder and, applying gentle pressure, work up toward the nape of your neck. Repeat on the other side.

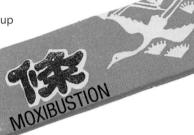

2. Follow the same line, but this time work in circular movements toward your hairline.

3. Massage from the spine along your waistline using firm outward movements.

4. Bend over with knees slightly bent and lightly pummel up and down your back with loose fists, keeping your wrists relaxed.

5. Hug yourself and feel around your shoulder blades for knots of tension, working up and down with your fingertips.

53 **Get on your knees when you next need to rest and relax your body** (this pose is also great for soothing a sore back). Kneel on the ground and, with arms by your sides, bend forward so that your head rests on the floor in front of you. Hold this position, breathing gently, for a couple of minutes and feel your knots unravel.

54 **For the ultimate in stressless living, spend a weekend outdoors with nature.** Take your watch off and wake up with the sun, go to sleep with the dark, and only eat when you're hungry. Limit distractions by unplugging the phone and hiding the TV remote control. Now you've only got yourself to entertain— just don't get stressed out about it.

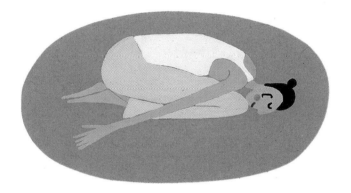

55 **Shiatsu is another kind of oriental medicine** which works on the meridians in your body to influence the flow of energy that runs through you (called *chi* in China and *ki* in Japan). A therapist will use careful pressure on receptive points, and may also knead tight muscles and rock your body to loosen stiff joints. Shiatsu is great for stress-related problems such as back and neck ache. Make sure you wear loose cotton clothing, as synthetic material may upset the energy flow.

56 **Do-It-Yourself Shiatsu**

Try these healing movements at home the next time your body is suffering from stress.

Head/Neck Aches:

Where? On the back of your hand, slide and press your finger along the bone between your thumb and first finger until you feel a small indentation and a sharp pain.

How? Press the flesh and rub firmly to release the pain, concentrating on the hand that feels the most sensitive.

Stress Relief:

Where? Slide your thumb between the bones of your middle and ring finger on your palm. When you reach the center of your palm, you should feel a slight ache.

How? Take a deep breath and press into your flesh deeply as you breathe out. Repeat on both hands.

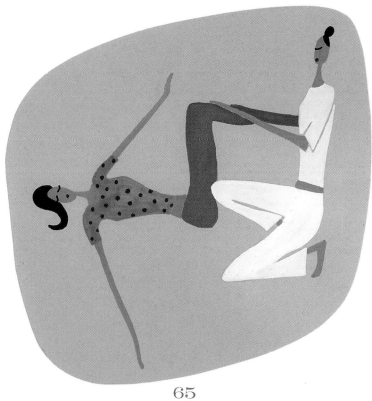

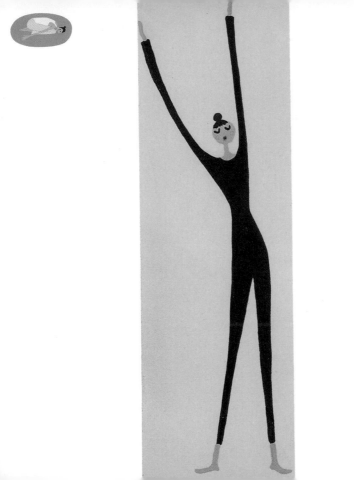

57 Stretching works like an internal massage, gently loosening tired, tense joints and muscles. Always stretch when your body is warm (cold muscles are too stiff) and breathe deeply throughout stretching exercises. This should be a pleasant experience that leaves you feeling relaxed, so if you feel pain at any time, stop. Simple but effective stretches include reaching for the sky, or lying on your back and stretching your arms and legs toward opposite sides of the room.

58 Get rid of tension by stroking your scalp. Start with your fingers on your eyebrows and run them upward through your hair and down the back of your head. Just five times should ease any frustration you feel.

59 **A stressed body could be in pain due to a past injury or bad posture.** Osteopathy and chiropractics can relieve the strain through manipulation and massage, and it's not all painful bone-crunching. The crack you hear as a therapist manipulates your body is due to air compression, not your bones breaking. Things may get a little tender as practitioners may prod tissues to test for tension, but this treatment is painless and pain-relieving.

60 **There's nothing like soaking your feet to distract yourself from your stressed-out head.** Fill a bowl with hot water that's just comfortable enough to stick your feet into. Add one tablespoon of sea salt or six drops of a relaxing essential oil (lavender, bergamot, marjoram, and sandalwood will do the job) and soak your feet and ankles for 15 minutes. Sleeping badly? Dunking your feet in this at night is also good for insomnia and can reduce the need to get up to pee in the night.

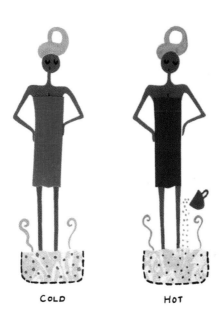

COLD   HOT

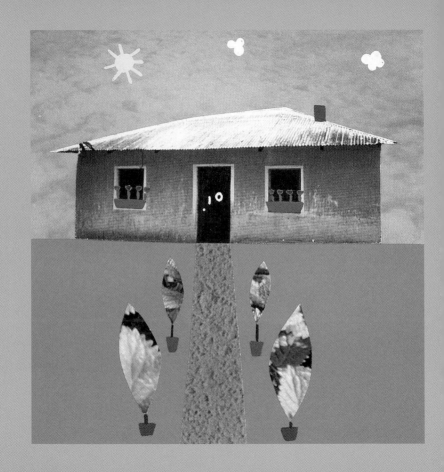

chapter 4

Home healing methods

61 If you're constantly searching for stuff in your purse, set a date to clean out the clutter in it. Organize your purse and you'll organize an important part of your daily life. Be ruthless. Do you really need to lug around six lipsticks when you always wear the same shade anyway?

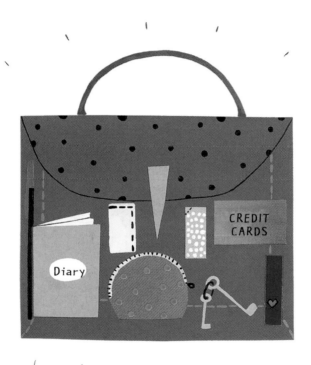

62 **Make a weekly chore positively pleasurable by adding a few drops of calming lavender oil to the water compartment of your iron.** Or fill up an atomizer with water and add six drops of lavender oil. Shake and spray onto your t-shirts before you iron them and the heat will release the aroma all around you.

63 **There are many ways to scent your surroundings with a relaxing aroma.** Buy a diffuser and burn your favorite oils to match the room to your mood. Pour a little water into the holder first and let it warm up before adding essential oil, and its scent will last longer.

64 **Buy a comfort cushion.** Some types of small beanbag pillows, filled with grain, can be heated in a microwave; they hold heat for an hour (read the label for guidelines). Sprinkle on six drops of a relaxing oil like lavender, chamomile, or marjoram, wrap the pillow around your neck, and unwind.

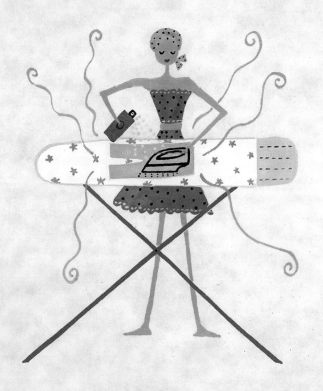

65 **There is no need to buy an expensive oil burner. For do-it-yourself diffusing, add a few drops of essential oil to small bowls of water and place them on radiators** or warm metal surfaces so the heat spreads the vapor. Or transform plain, cheap candles into room diffusers. Light the wick and allow a puddle of wax to collect around the top. Then sprinkle on six drops of relaxing essential oil and the wax will be just the right temperature to release the aroma.

66 **Buy candles in a wide range of colors and light the one that suits your mood:**

- *White*—cleanses
- *Orange*—lifts your spirits
- *Pink*—wakes you up
- *Red*—sparks passion
- *Green*—soothes nerves.

67 **Make a cozy, roaring log fire even more restful**—add a few drops of essential oil to a log. Leave to soak in for 30 minutes, and then set it alight.

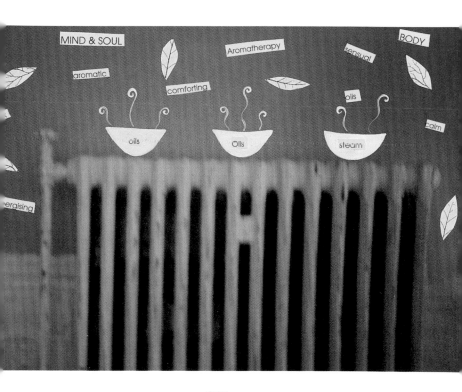

68 Color can seriously affect your mood, so make sure you surround yourself with the right shades. The dull colors we often choose in winter (like black, navy and brown) only add to the depression of winter's long dark days and nights, but switch to a bright color and feel your gloomy mood lift immediately.

69 Feeling lethargic? Then wearing red will give you a lift, but, if you're already agitated, it will just add to your anger. Being a warming color, red can also ease aches and pains, like backache. If you wake up irritable, green will calm your nerves, while blue and violet are healing shades. Wear yellow to expand your mind.

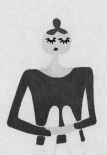

70 Most of us spend the day under outdated fluorescent strip lighting, but scientists have discovered that people deprived of full-spectrum light (i.e. light that simulates all the colors of natural daylight) suffer more fatigue, decreased performance, lowered immune defenses, headaches, and depression. If you're feeling stressed, angry, upset, or depressed, entering a room with conventional lighting will make your mood worse, but a room with full-spectrum light will have an instant calming effect. Fill your home with relaxing rays by investing in full-spectrum or daylight-simulating light bulbs.

71 Color in the home.
Blue will keep you cool in a hot steamy kitchen and green will calm your nerves when cooking. Avoid red, which only adds to the already heated atmosphere. Violet is the perfect bedroom color as it relaxes and eases insomnia. But avoid too-bright curtains, which can cause sleeping problems; go for soft, pastel shades instead. For your main living area, choose green, which will calm your mind and body and soothe away the day's exhaustion, or indigo, which will encourage a positive frame of mind and push away negative thoughts.

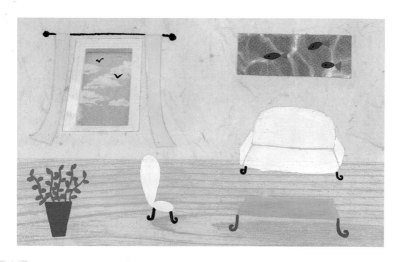

72 You may not be able to change the decor of your office, but you can add color to your desk to help you through the day. If you're bored, orange will help bring you to life. Green is perfect if you suffer from nerves, and blue will calm stressful situations. Avoid red, as it agitates atmospheres, and too much yellow hinders concentration.

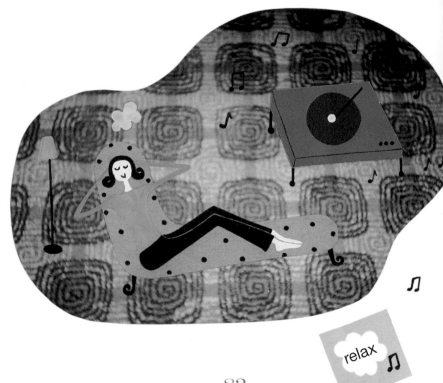

82

relax

73 Music can improve your mood, however ugly your surroundings. Different frequencies of sound affect the body in different ways. High frequencies stimulate the central nervous system and low frequencies (i.e. most popular music) can deplete energy. Apparently, the music of Mozart contains the most perfectly balanced harmonies, so close your eyes and go classical.

74 Make yourself an anti-stress scent by adding six drops of lavender oil, four drops of sandalwood, four drops of bergamot and four drops of chamomile to four ounces of vegetable oil (any oil in your larder will do). Then use to massage, as a body oil, or add to your bath water.

75 When you're feeling stressed out, check your jaw. Chances are it's locked solid. Release the tension by moving your lower jaw from side to side, or reach for some raw vegetables. The crunching motion will instantly unclamp you.

76 A bouquet of flowers can change the mood of a room. Choose blue to cool the atmosphere on a hot day and a green plant such as ivy or yucca to bring you a sense of peace.

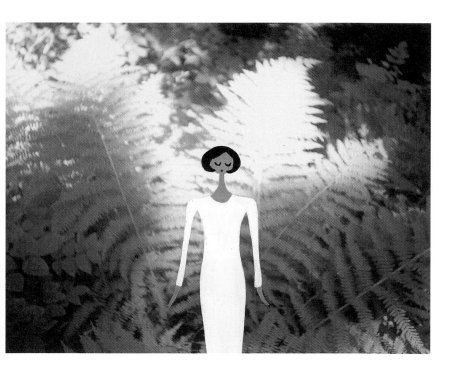

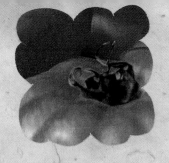

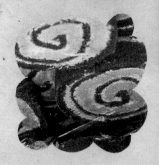

77 Food doesn't just taste good; it can make you feel good too. The right meal can pick you up when you're feeling depressed, or calm you down when you're feeling stressed. Nutritionists now know that the natural chemicals in food can change the way you feel by influencing the chemicals in your brain. Feeling lethargic? Eat meat, fish, or poultry, which all make you more alert. Need soothing at the end of a stressful day? Choose pasta, bread, potatoes, rice or grains. Feeling down? Sweet foods encourage your body to release mood-improving endorphins. An excuse (if one is needed) to fill up your refrigerator in times of trouble.

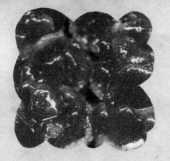

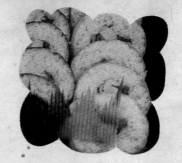

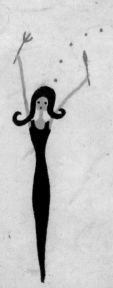

78 Feeling anxious? Then eat an apple. The scent has been found to fend off nervous feelings, especially when mixed with cinnamon. Sprinkle some on your apple before eating and prepare to feel peaceful.

79 Feng Shui the front of your house and feel a burst of energy every time you come home. If you have to battle with a broken lock or pass through a neglected garden, life will seem more of a struggle. But make your entrance welcoming and you'll feel an instant boost. Plant flowers or invest in a couple of window boxes. Paint a hallway red or orange so that it will exude warm, cozy vibes. And if your house has two or more numbers, position the second one slightly higher than the first to give you a lift every time you walk through your door. A tidy home means a tidy mind. Get rid of unnecessary clutter and take it to a charity. Very rewarding.

80 Move the TV out of your bedroom. Rays emitted from a television can affect your nervous system and stop you from sleeping soundly. Curl up with a good book instead.

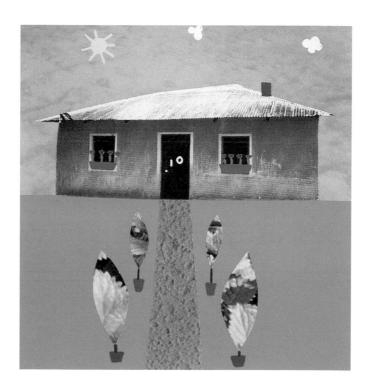

89

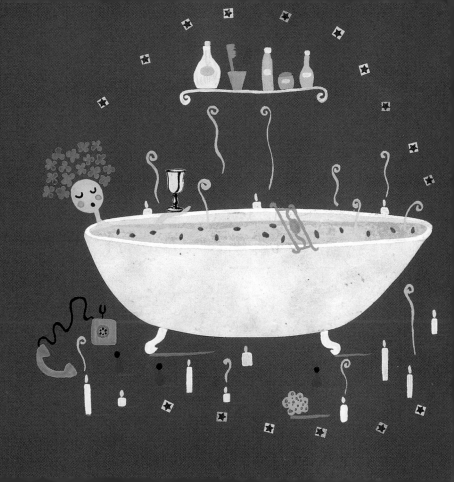

chapter 5

Day-to-day destressers

81 Go out in the backyard for instant stress relief. Plant-filled spaces have been proven to relax the mind and provide a peaceful sanctuary away from a chaotic world. And if your garden is large enough, the level of pollutants there will be lower than average too. Plants can also prove worthwhile at work. Research shows they absorb common pollutants and pump out water to counteract low humidity in air-conditioned offices. And some plants can also soak up sound waves, which is why they're used alongside busy roads to shield local houses from high noise levels. Your office may not be built on a highway, but surrounding yourself with plant life may help insulate you from the noisy conversations of co-workers.

82 Set up a special place in your home where you can retreat when things go wrong. Stick up your favorite photos of friends and family, and set out significant souvenirs you've collected over the years. Then, when you're feeling stressed out, you can sit in your shrine surrounded by all your best memories—and remember.

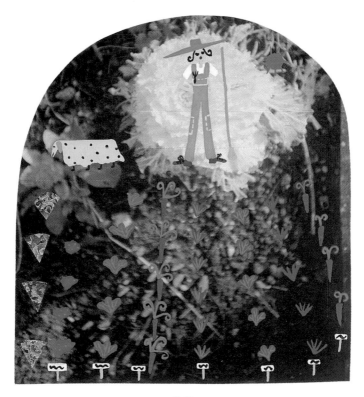

83 Find time for the things you enjoy, whether it's visiting a quiet art gallery or going on an expensive shopping spree. If it helps you forget your problems, then anything you love doing can be a success.

 Five-Minute Stress Fixers:

- *Eat something you love*
- *Be nice to someone*
- *Pet an animal*
- *Plan a trip away from home*
- *Do a good deed.*

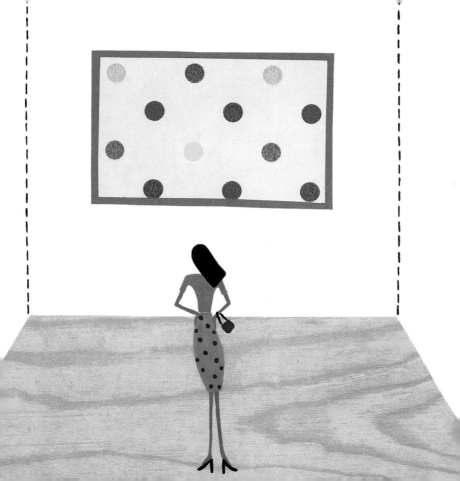

85 Fresh air is fashionable. Oxygen bars began in Tokyo, Japan, and have since spread to other smog-filled cities such as Hong Kong and the home of clean living, Los Angeles. Hollywood celebrities swear by this latest fix, which uses a state-of-the-art nasal cannula to pump out 95% concentrated oxygen. In just a few minutes, manufacturers promise you'll feel revitalized and be able to concentrate better. We think a hobby that gets you outdoors is better. Choose something like birdwatching and you'll get in touch with nature while learning something new—it's also a great way to relieve stressful thoughts.

86 Learn to manage your time more effectively, and each day won't seem such a struggle. Plan your work day and prioritize what needs to be done. Set aside time for outgoing phonecalls and try to be brief. Tackle one task at a time and, whenever possible, handle each piece of paper only once. Be prepared for meetings, and allow extra time for travel, in order to avoid arriving in a state of panic.

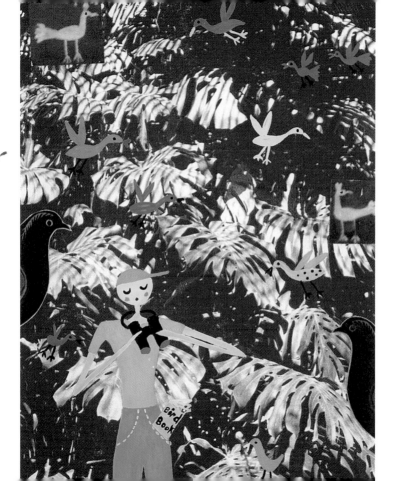

87 **Stress forces you to take shallow breaths, which don't let your body get rid of tension the way a deep breath can.** Most of us only use 30% of our breathing capacity, a habit picked up in childhood when we were taught to hold in our stomachs. A large lung full of air centers and calms you (which is why actors practice deep breathing before they go onstage), and also boosts your immune system. Practice this breathing exercise the next time you're out walking. To a count of four, breathe in through your nose right down into your stomach, hold for one, and then push the breath out again for a count of four. Don't worry if you feel a bit light-headed—it just means your body's not used to taking in such a deep breath of oxygen.

88 **Ready to blow your top?** When you're stressed out, your adrenal glands go into overdrive and you need to put on the brakes. The best way to do this is with some deep breathing. Roll your eyes upward and close them, then breathe deeply and slowly to a count of ten. Now isn't that better?

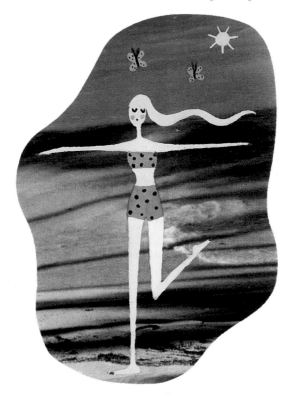

99

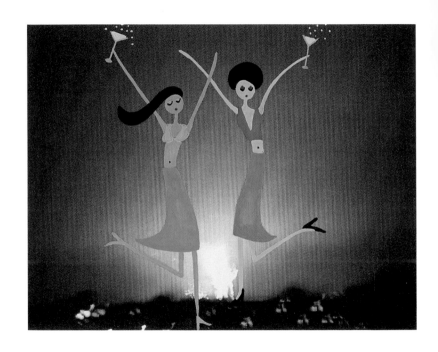

89 **Stored stress won't stand a chance against a good party.** The right music can lift the lowest spirits, and dancing till dawn releases tight, tense muscles. A tipple or two will also help you shed your inhibitions and make you feel relaxed, talkative and feeling great. But don't overdo things or you will feel far from great the next morning.

90 **Laughter is good for you.** It relaxes tense muscles, eases tiredness, and triggers the release of "feel-good" hormones in your brain. It even helps fight off infection. Got no reason to giggle? Then watch a funny film, read a witty book, or arrange to see an upbeat friend. Whatever you choose to do, if it feels good, it'll be doing you good.

91 Recipe for a stress-busting bath:

1. Make the water warm, not hot, which would overstimulate your senses.

2. Add a few drops of relaxing essential oil after the water has finished running. Sandalwood is especially good for calming and relaxing a hassled head, and is also moisturizing dry skin.

3. Light candles and dim the lights —candlelight is much easier on the eyes than electric lightbulbs.

4. Shut the door to keep people out and the relaxing vapors in.

5. Unplug the phone and turn on some soothing music, which will block out other sounds and help slow down a racing mind.

6. Lie back, close your eyes, and breathe deeply to inhale the essential oil vapors and induce relaxation.

7. Beginning at the top of your head, relax every muscle in your body from your scalp right down to the tips of your toes.

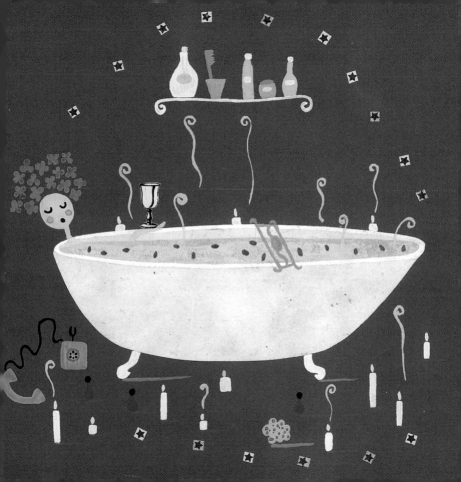

92 **A good massage is literally hands-on healing.** All that kneading and stroking stimulates lymphatic drainage, which gets rid of toxins from the body. The result? Tension is eased, sore muscles soothed, and emotional stress released. And a relaxed body works better with deeper breathing and improved digestion. There are many types of massage, from deep pressure for dispersing knots to holistic healing for stored emotional stress. Talk to your therapist beforehand to ensure you're getting the right massage for your muscles.

93 **Essential oils that promise to calm stress produce slower frequency brain waves to quieten your mind,** and many also have anti-depressant properties. Ones to choose at the end of a tough day include:

- *Bergamot—helps anxiety*
- *Chamomile—eases tension*
- *Lavender—balances emotions*
- *Mandarin—gently sedates*
- *Peppermint—calms nerves*
- *Rose—helps with grief*
- *Rosewood—relieves stress.*

Use them in your bath, in a vaporizer, or mixed with a base oil for a great massage.

104

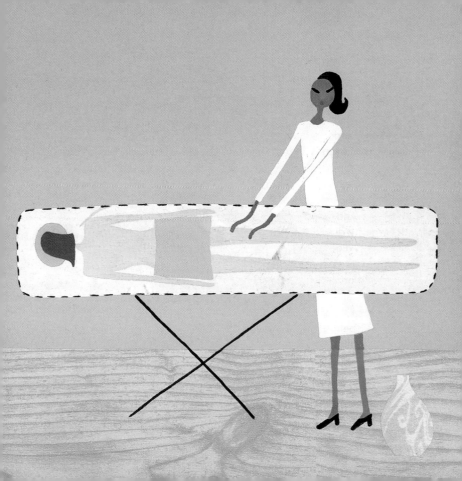

94 **Many of us live in cities where buildings are getting taller, with the result that we get less natural light than ever before.** But humans evolved in balance with the natural cycles of night and day, and a lack of light can literally throw your body out of rhythm. In skyscraper cities, high levels of violent crime have even been linked to perpetrators having a lack of sunlight. To control your own mood swings, spend more time outdoors, even on cloudy days. Walking a dog is great exercise and will make the most laid-back animal love you for life. If you don't have one of your own, walk your neighbors. He'll be glad of the extra time in bed.

95 **Missed the bus? Boss shouting again?** Take in a deep breath and mentally push out all the pain with one big exhalation of air.

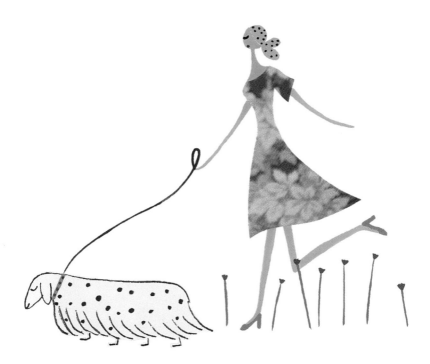

96 **Reading demands concentration** (unlike watching the TV). The result is that you completely turn yourself off from the stressful world around you. Make time for reading and escape into your chosen fantasy world for a while.

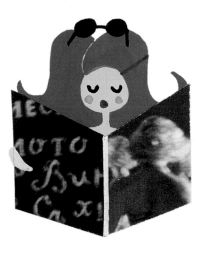

97 Constant mental stimulation can be stressful. Spend a few minutes each day doing absolutely nothing in total peace and quiet. Don't talk, read, watch TV, or listen to music. Just be.

98 Singing or humming can relieve stress, as it produces relaxing vibrations in your throat. Just make sure you're not stressing anyone else out with your tune.

99 **If stress makes you bite your nails, pull your hair or pick your skin, buy a stress ball.** It is far less offensive than fiddling with yourself.

100 **Going through a rough time?** Then pamper your body with pleasures you would normally deny yourself. Having your hair done is a major morale booster (if you look good, you'll feel better), and even if you only have time for a quick blow-dry, you'll leave the salon less stressed out.

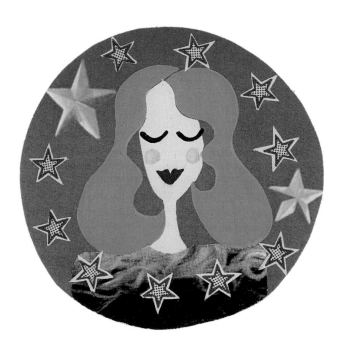

An AOL Time Warner Company

Printed in China
First printing: 10 9 8 7 6 5 4 3 2 1

Library of Congress Control Number: 2001097171

ISBN: 1-931722-07-2